TRISOMY 18
NEW AND EXPECTANT PARENT RESOURCE GUIDE

First published by Support Organization for Trisomy 18, 13, and Other Related Disorders (SOFT), 2024
Copyright © 2024 SOFT

First edition.

ISBN: 979-8-9914465-0-1

Cover design by Jen Gilmore
Typeset by Jen Gilmore

TO ALL THE CHILDREN
AND FAMILIES IMPACTED
BY TRISOMY 18

TABLE OF CONTENTS

INTRODUCTION:

The purpose of this book is to assist the expectant family that has received a possible or confirmed diagnosis of trisomy 18 (Edwards syndrome). This book will help you understand your pregnancy, the related decisions, and will be a guide for you throughout your pregnancy, and at the time of birth. We have bolded terms throughout the book that are also defined in the Glossary.

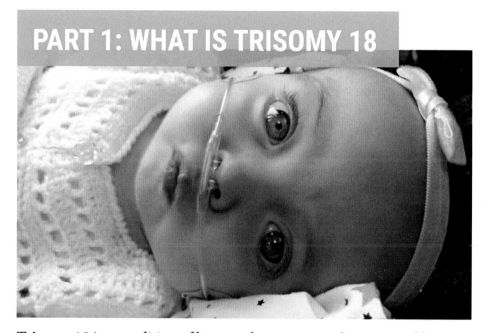

PART 1: WHAT IS TRISOMY 18

Trisomy 18 is a condition of human chromosomes that is caused by an extra or third 18th chromosome, hence trisomy 18. This extra 18th chromosome leads to a specific pattern of physical findings known as the trisomy 18 **syndrome**, also known as **Edwards syndrome**. **(NOTE: genetic testing before or after birth must be done to confirm the diagnosis.)**

Trisomy 18 has an impact on the health of the children who have the condition. It includes three major implications: the occurrence of medically important birth defects (especially of the heart), a higher than expected frequency of infant mortality making it a potentially life-limiting condition, and a developmental disability in older infants and children.

The actual reason or cause of the extra 18th chromosome is not known even after years of research. There is no way to have prevented its occurrence prior to conception, and there is nothing you could have avoided or done to stop it from happening.

"I received the diagnosis at 12 weeks. My first thought was what in the world is T18? Took a moment to process my emotions, and cried because of what was told to me about T18."

There are three types of chromosome findings seen in persons with the trisomy 18 syndrome. Approximately 95% will have a full or complete trisomy 18 (see Figure 1) in all body cells. The remainder (about 5% of infants) will have a partial trisomy, an extra piece of the 18 **chromosome** due to a rearrangement of part of the chromosome (usually attached to another chromosome, called a **translocation**), or have **mosaicism** (a mixture of two different cell populations, usually some normal cells and some trisomy 18 cells).

Chromosome study showing trisomy 18

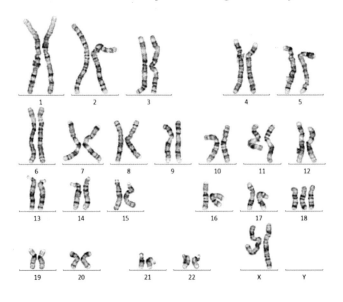

Note the 23 pairs of numbered chromosomes with chromosome 18 having 3 (trisomy) rather than 2 chromosomes.

Figure 1: karyotype figure provided courtesy of Dr Erica Anderson, ARUP Laboratories

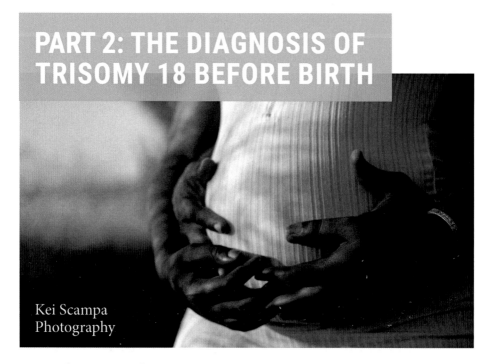

PART 2: THE DIAGNOSIS OF TRISOMY 18 BEFORE BIRTH

Kei Scampa
Photography

Prenatal testing to detect trisomy 18 can be divided into two basic groups: screening tests and diagnostic tests. Screening tests include quadruple screen, **noninvasive prenatal screening or testing (NIPS or NIPT)** , and ultrasound. These tests do not make a definitive diagnosis of trisomy 18.

The quadruple screen is an older test, requires a blood sample from the mother, and looks at specific hormones and proteins.

The NIPS or NIPT (cell-free DNA) test is a newer screening test that also requires a blood sample from the mother. This test looks for fetal DNA fragments that have crossed the placenta and are in the mother's bloodstream. The fetal DNA in the mothers serum is measured. This test is typically offered at 10 weeks or later. While almost all fetuses who have full trisomy 18 will show the excess DNA, not all fetuses with a positive result will have Edwards syndrome. It is important to ask the doctor or genetic counselor how likely it is that a positive result predicts Edward syndrome (**positive predictive value PPV**).

An **ultrasound** can be used in the first trimester to look for extra fluid and thickness at the back of the fetus' neck. This type of ultrasound is typically performed by a maternal fetal medicine specialist (MFM). If there is extra fluid or thickness, this can be a sign of a chromosomal abnormality. An ultrasound during the second or third trimester of pregnancy can be used to look at the fetus' organs and various structures between 18-22 weeks. Findings such as suspected heart defects, brain or spine abnormalities, and rocker bottom feet could be associated with trisomy 18 and may lead to your care provider suggesting further ultrasounds or diagnostic testing. Many of the physical findings seen on prenatal ultrasound are not medically important but provide clues to the diagnosis before birth (or in the newborn period). These can include: prominence to the back part of the head, small mouth and jaw, short breastbone, and clenched fist with index finger overlapping the third.

> "I panicked, started googling and it was a super emotional rollercoaster. I called my family members, no one understood and thought it wasn't real and test wasn't accurate."

Since quadruple screen, NIPS or NIPT, and ultrasound are screening tests, a definitive diagnosis prenatally requires diagnostic testing. Diagnostic tests include **chorionic villus sampling (CVS)** at 10-12 weeks or **amniocentesis** at 15-16 weeks. Both are considered invasive tests and have less than 1% of pregnancy loss over normal risk for pregnancy loss.

CVS is performed in the first trimester, and involves taking a small sample of the developing placenta for the study. Due to this, CVS carries a slightly higher risk than amniocentesis. The benefit of CVS is that the procedure is performed earlier in pregnancy, and thus the result is back sooner (12-13 weeks of pregnancy compared to 16-17 weeks for an amniocentesis). Knowing early is important for families who would consider termination, as abortion laws are changing rapidly and are becoming increasingly more restrictive depending on the state (see Part 9).

Amniocentesis can be performed anytime after 15 weeks, and involves obtaining a sample of the fluid surrounding the developing fetus. Both the CVS and amniocentesis use ultrasound to guide the needle during sampling. These tests are most often performed by maternal-fetal medicine (MFM) specialists, or "high-risk OB's." While there are rare exceptions, CVS and amniocentesis are generally considered very accurate. Risks of both procedures include miscarriage, premature rupture of membranes, infection, or bleeding from the placenta; however, these are typically very rare.

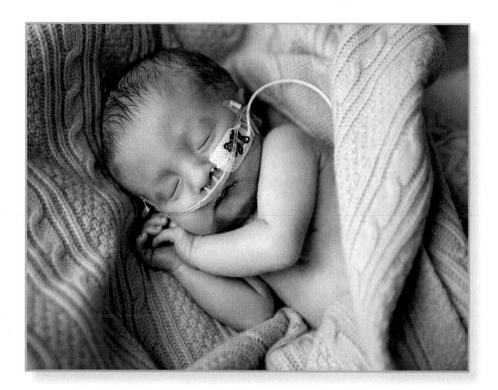

PART 3: OTHER TESTS DURING PREGNANCY

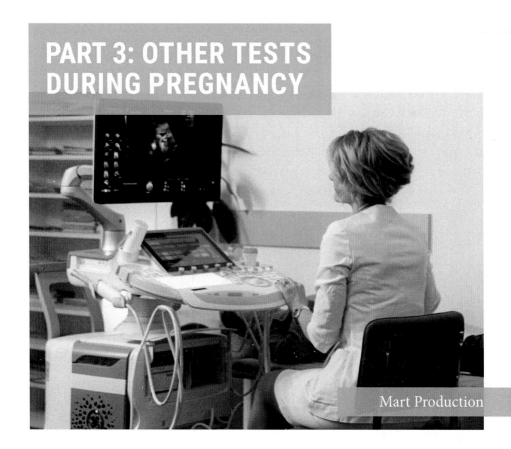

Mart Production

Once the diagnosis of trisomy 18 is confirmed, the need for additional monitoring and testing during the pregnancy is offered to assist in providing the best possible outcome for both the mother and baby. This section will explain what these tests are and why they are performed.

If a genetic difference is suspected, the pregnancy is typically considered a high risk pregnancy, and will be followed by both a general obstetrician-gynecologist (Ob-Gyn) and a maternal-fetal medicine (MFM) specialist. They can perform the ultrasound mentioned above looking for changes in the organs (often called a "level 2 ultrasound"). Heart defects are commonly associated with trisomy 18, and they may either perform or recommend a special heart ultrasound of the fetus called a fetal **echocardiogram**.

A fetal echocardiogram evaluates the anatomy and function of the chambers of the heart. This test is typically done after 20 weeks gestation and looks for various heart defects such as ventricular septal defects (VSD), or other more complex cardiac defects (see Part 4). This specialized ultrasound will look at how the blood flows through the heart and vessels leading to and from the heart. The images from the echocardiogram will be interpreted by pediatric cardiologists (see Part 5) and MFMs to help determine what, if any, treatments need to be considered following birth. This echocardiogram may be performed again during pregnancy, or once the baby is born.

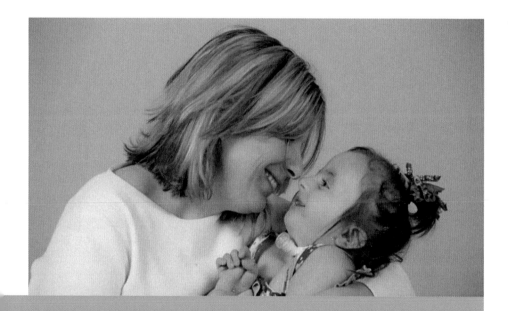

"At first I was so frightened of Kari! She seemed more "abnormal" than "normal" so I didn't act normal. But, when I finally realized that Kari had the same needs as every other child, I let go of my fears and began to embrace every opportunity to love her. She was a sweet and loving young girl who touched hearts by simply being herself!"

There are a number of other complications that can arise during pregnancy. **Fetuses** (babies inside the womb) with trisomy 18 are at an increased risk for miscarriage and stillbirth. The risk for the loss during pregnancy decreases as the pregnancy progresses.

Some mothers may require additional testing in the third trimester of pregnancy. These tests are typically performed along with fetal growth ultrasounds done every 3 to 4 weeks in the third trimester. They may include: fetal non-stress testing (NST), measurement of the fluid around the baby (amniotic fluid indexes, or AFI), and/or a biophysical profile (BPP). Each office has their own protocol for performing these tests.

+ Non-stress test: Monitors are placed on the mother's abdomen to record contractions as well as the baby's heart beats. This test typically takes between 20 and 60 minutes.

+ Amniotic fluid index (AFI): Ultrasonographic measurement of the fluid around the baby. Pregnancies complicated by genetic conditions are often associated with fluid abnormalities. This is performed to look at how the placenta is performing, how well the baby is swallowing, as well as making and voiding urine.

+ Biophysical profile (BPP): Completed during an ultrasound and looks at the baby's heart rate, breathing, movement, muscle tone, and the amount of amniotic fluid around the baby. This test can be done after 28 weeks.

Other more specialized ultrasounds can be performed if there is concern for problems with growth. Umbilical cord dopplers are used to evaluate how well the blood flows from the placenta to the baby. They may also be performed more frequently depending on other ultrasound findings or growth problems.

The OB/GYNs and MFMs will use these third trimester tests to help determine the best timing of delivery. More concerning findings may warrant earlier delivery; however, otherwise uncomplicated pregnancies may be able to continue until closer to your due date. Multiple factors go into the timing of delivery, and this is a discussion that should occur with your care provider.

PART 4: WHAT DOES TRISOMY 18 MEAN FOR YOUR BABY AND FAMILY?

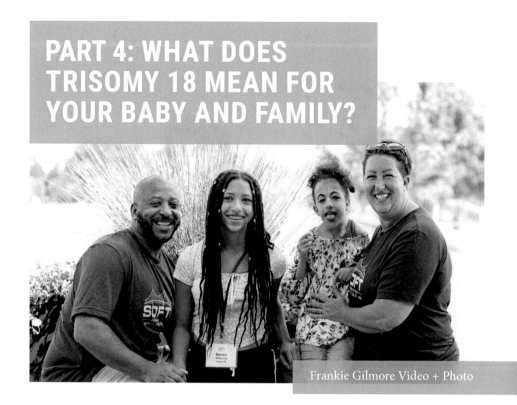

Frankie Gilmore Video + Photo

"The day he was at school using his Tobii communication device and he said "I love you", "I am happy" to me when we were on Zoom. I started to cry, and all his teachers and support staff teared up with joy."

As mentioned in Part 1, trisomy 18 is sometimes referred to as Edwards syndrome, named for the British doctor who first described the condition. It includes the occurrence of medically important birth defects. We will discuss the birth defects and other medical issues in this section.

Birth Defects
Almost all children born with trisomy 18 will have **birth defects** (the medical term is congenital malformations); however, each child is different, and the occurrence of these individual challenges is highly variable. The most common and important problem is a defect of the heart. About 90% of children with trisomy 18 will have a heart malformation. The actual defect varies, but the most common include:

Ventricular septal defect (VSD): an opening between the lower chambers of the heart which prevents the heart from pumping blood correctly (a heart murmur is generally heard from this finding)

Atrial septal defect (ASD): an opening between the two upper chambers of the heart making it difficult for the heart to pump sufficient oxygen-rich blood to body tissues (a heart murmur is often heard)

Patent ductus arteriosus (PDA): a heart defect involving a persistent opening of the channel between two major blood vessels leaving the heart. This is normal during pregnancy, but this channel usually closes near the time of birth. Lack of closure can contribute to pulmonary hypertension (discussed below)

In addition, children with trisomy 18 often have a change of one or two of the four heart valves. This combination is referred to as a ventricular septal defect with polyvalvular dysplasia. If there is blockage of the pulmonic valve, then the combination may be called tetralogy of Fallot.

The majority of heart lesions are usually not those that cause major problems in the newborn period (first 4 weeks of life). But sometimes, the heart defect in combination with respiratory issues, can lead to breathing difficulties and heart issues in the first two weeks of life. Only about 1 in 6 of children with trisomy 18 will have a more complicated or serious heart defect noted before or soon after birth. These heart defects include a double outlet right ventricle (DORV) and hypoplastic left heart syndrome (HLHS). The potential option for heart surgery should be discussed with the specialists prenatally and in the newborn period.

Other Medical Issues

Along with cardiac defects, the next most common medically important conditions associated with trisomy 18 are respiratory-related concerns. Respiratory difficulties include:

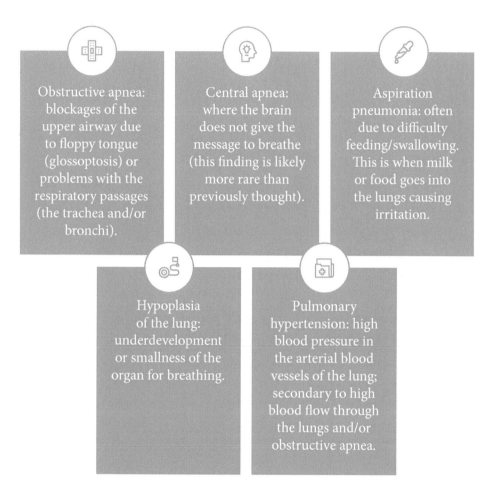

Obstructive apnea: blockages of the upper airway due to floppy tongue (glossoptosis) or problems with the respiratory passages (the trachea and/or bronchi).

Central apnea: where the brain does not give the message to breathe (this finding is likely more rare than previously thought).

Aspiration pneumonia: often due to difficulty feeding/swallowing. This is when milk or food goes into the lungs causing irritation.

Hypoplasia of the lung: underdevelopment or smallness of the organ for breathing.

Pulmonary hypertension: high blood pressure in the arterial blood vessels of the lung; secondary to high blood flow through the lungs and/or obstructive apnea.

Because of the various challenges and differences, older infants and children are followed by the medical specialists who are experts in the particular problem. These specialists are usually located at children's hospitals. Your primary care provider can make referrals to the appropriate medical center for you (see Part 5). Some hospitals have comprehensive care teams that help organize the care of children with medically complex conditions.

Other common birth defects and conditions seen in trisomy 18 (Edwards syndrome) and their estimated frequency include:

- Esophageal atresia, blockage of the esophagus with or without a connection to the trachea (windpipe) - 5-10%

- Spina bifida (opening in the back from a defect in the spine) - 5%

- Diaphragmatic hernia - 5%

- Radial aplasia (small or missing radial bone of forearm and thumb) - 5-10%

- Physical defects of the shape and position kidneys -50% (but usually not a major medical problem)

- Cleft lip with or without cleft palate - 5-10% (lack of closure of the upper lip and roof of the mouth)

- Seizures - about 25-30% of infants and young children develop a seizure condition, occasionally in the newborn but usually later in childhood

- Feeding difficulties/challenges in the ability to breast or bottle feed, sometimes referred to as dysphagia-very common

- Developmental disabilities - significant limitation in the development of skills such as sitting, walking, and speaking are present in all children

PART 5: SPECIALISTS AND TEAMS

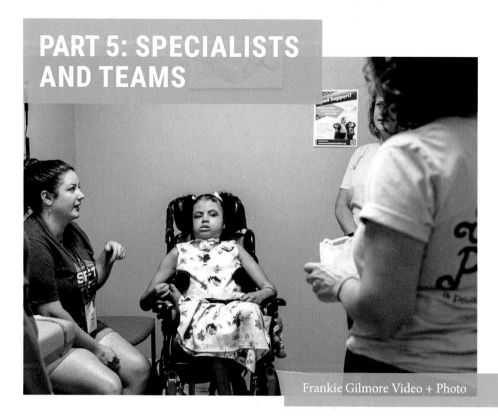

Frankie Gilmore Video + Photo

Now that your baby has been found to have features associated with Edwards syndrome, your medical team may expand to include a number of specialists who can provide further diagnosis of current or potential medical needs as well as treatment options. Parents often find it can be helpful to engage a number of these specialists before the baby is born (prenatally). Additionally, some communities have Fetal Centers where families might be referred.

A **Fetal Center** is often based at a children's hospital and provides teams of specialists making access to the appropriate professionals easier for parents. The number of fetal centers in the U.S. has increased over recent years. A current list can be found at fetalhealthfoundation.org/treatment-centers/

"Trisomy is an amplified version of why we go into medicine in the first place. There is a group of people that you can develop the capability to help."

Prenatal Consults:

Prenatal consults can help parents better understand the capabilities and care provided at the hospital where you are delivering, and may help determine where you deliver your baby. Please keep in mind that consultations with some of the health care professionals listed below will be dependent on the ultrasound findings seen on the prenatal ultrasounds. Most families will consult with a neonatologist, an obstetrician and/or MFM specialist, a geneticist or genetic counselor, and a palliative care professional. If the baby has a heart defect, then meeting with the pediatric cardiologist and possibly the heart surgeon is important. If the baby has spina bifida, meeting with the pediatric neurosurgeon can be helpful.

- Obstetrician/Gynecologist (OB/GYN) - a physician who specializes in maternal health. They will be the primary physician during the pregnancy and will be responsible for directing and managing routine OB appointments, labor/delivery admission, and will most often perform the delivery. They may 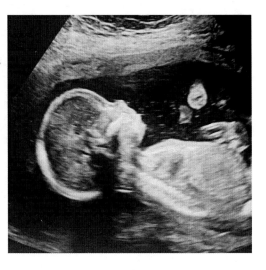 also work with certified nurse midwives (CNMs) who may also be involved in the prenatal care/delivery. After medical school, training for an OB/GYN includes four years of residency in obstetrics/gynecology.

- Maternal Fetal Medicine (MFM) - a physician who specializes in taking care of high risk mothers and babies with medical issues primarily during their pregnancy. This doctor will likely be the first doctor you are referred to by your primary OB/GYN. They will help manage your pregnancy and provide recommendations regarding monitoring as well as delivery. After medical school, their training includes four years of residency in obstetrics and gynecology (OB/GYN) followed by a three-year fellowship.

(+) Medical Geneticist -
a physician who specializes in the evaluation, diagnosis, management, treatment, and counseling of individuals with inherited disease. After medical school, they usually complete an integrated residency program of two years of internal medicine, pediatrics or OB/GYN followed by two years of medical genetics; some train in a specialty like pediatrics and then complete a two-year categorical residency in medical genetics and genomics.

(+) Genetic Counselor -
a healthcare professional who is trained in medical genetics and counseling. Certified genetic counselors work closely with physicians in OB/GYN, MFM, and medical genetics. They are very knowledgeable in genetic testing and genetic conditions.

(+) Pediatric Cardiologist -
a pediatrician that specializes in taking care of children with problems of the heart's structure and rhythm. They can look at your baby's heart before they are born by fetal echocardiogram (ultrasound of the heart) or MRI. They often work with pediatric cardiothoracic surgeons for planning regarding surgical repair of a heart defect. After medical school, their training includes three years of residency in general pediatrics followed by three years of fellowship in pediatric cardiology.

(+) Pediatric Cardiothoracic Surgeon -
a surgeon who specializes in taking care of children (and some adults) with serious heart or lung conditions that require surgical intervention. It may be helpful to meet with this specialist prior to delivery depending on the specific heart defect and/or your geographic location. After medical school, their training includes five years of residency in general surgery followed by 2-3 years cardiothoracic surgery fellowship followed by an additional 2-4 years fellowship in pediatric cardiothoracic surgery.

(+) Neonatalogist -
a pediatrician who specializes in the care of newborn infants, especially those who are ill or born early. They work in the Neonatal Intensive Care Unit (NICU). You can meet with them prior to your

delivery to help set up a care plan for your child and also find out the type of care they will provide to your child. After medical school, their training includes three years of residency in general pediatrics followed by a three-year fellowship in neonatal care.

- ⊕ Pediatrician - a primary care physician who specializes in taking care of children. It is important that this doctor is comfortable taking care of children with complex medical needs. After medical school, their training includes three years of residency in general pediatrics.

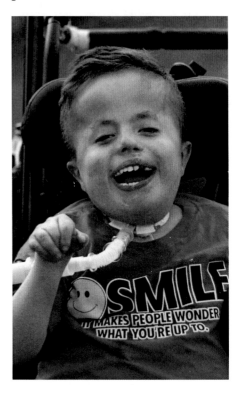

- ⊕ Palliative care specialist - physician or nurse with special training who provides support and guidance for families whose baby has a potential life-limiting condition such as trisomy 18 (Edwards syndrome). These specialists support families in decision making both prenatally and after birth. A palliative care physician's training includes a residency in another area, like pediatrics, and a fellowship in palliative medicine.

Postnatal Consults:
Depending on your baby's medical needs, you may meet with additional specialists after your baby is delivered. These postnatal consults can happen in the hospital or after discharge. Based on your child's changing needs, additional specialists may become part of your care team throughout your child's life. For other resources regarding physicians who may be part of your child's team, visit https://www.healthychildren.org/English/family-life/health-management/pediatric-specialists/Pages/default.aspx

⊕ Pediatric Surgeon -
a surgeon who specializes in treating newborns, infants, children, and teens. They may also meet with you before your baby is born if there are conditions that can be treated while in the womb or will need surgery immediately after birth. After medical school, their training includes five years of general surgery residency followed by a two-year fellowship in pediatric surgery.

⊕ Pediatric Pulmonologist -
a pediatrician who specializes in treating children with breathing problems and lung diseases. They manage conditions such as asthma, cystic fibrosis, and complex airways/lung disease that require ventilators and other breathing equipment. After medical school, their training includes three years of residency in general pediatrics followed by a three-year fellowship in pediatric pulmonology.

⊕ Pediatric Neurologist -
a pediatrician who specializes in treating children that have problems with their nervous system. This includes the brain, spinal cord, nerves, and muscles. They also have different tests like EEG that they can use to help look at electrical activity in the brain. After medical school, their training includes a combined child neurology residency program of two years of general pediatrics and three years of child neurology.

⊕ Pediatric Neurosurgeon -
a surgeon who specializes in children with birth defects or diseases

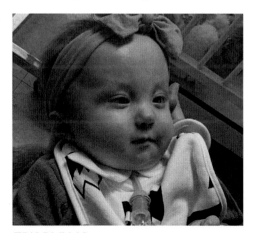

of their brain, spinal cord, nerves, and muscles such as spina bifida, Chiari malformations, and other conditions that can be associated with trisomy 18 (Edwards syndrome). Depending on the condition, they may continue management of the condition into adulthood. After medical school, their training includes one year of general surgery followed by five or more years of neurosurgical residency with an additional year of training in pediatric neurosurgery.

(+) Pediatric Otolaryngologist (ENT) -
a surgeon who specializes in treating diseases of the ears, nose, throat and upper airway. They perform surgeries such as ear tubes and tracheostomy placements, as well as, have cameras that look into these areas to look at anatomy. They play an important role in the assessment for potential hearing loss in trisomy 18 (Edwards syndrome). After medical school, they complete one year of general surgery training followed by four years of ENT residency and one-year fellowship in pediatric ENT.

(+) Pediatric Orthopedic Surgeon -
a surgeon who specializes in children who have bone deformities or broken bones. After medical school, they complete a five-year residency in orthopedics followed by a one-year fellowship in pediatric orthopedics and/or pediatric spinal deformity.

(+) Pediatric Gastroenterologist -
a pediatrician who specializes in children with diseases of the gastrointestinal tract, liver, and nutritional issues. This includes food allergies, difficulty swallowing, feeding, constipation, and problems with the pancreas or intestines. They can also perform procedures like placing feeding tubes and using cameras to look at anatomy. After medical school, they complete a three-year pediatric residency followed by a three-year fellowship in gastroenterology.

(+) Comprehensive Care Teams -
an established team of specialists who work together with the goal of providing better communication among team members and with families. These specialized teams are available at some children's hospitals, and some hospitals in the U.S. are establishing teams specifically for the care of children with trisomy conditions (see Weaver in References).

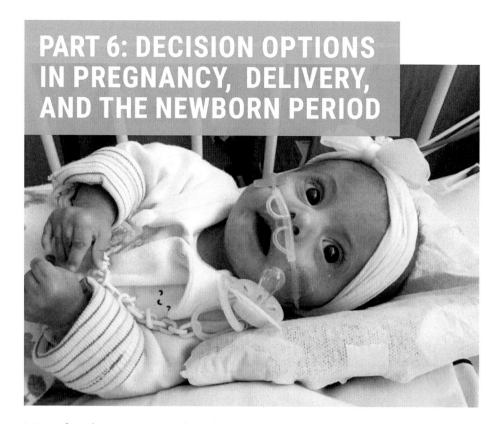

PART 6: DECISION OPTIONS IN PREGNANCY, DELIVERY, AND THE NEWBORN PERIOD

Many families question what options they have and how to make decisions regarding their pregnancy after receiving a diagnosis of trisomy 18. There is no correct answer for this, just what is correct for your family and your baby.

After the diagnosis is made during pregnancy, families will face the hard decision to either continue or terminate the pregnancy (see Part 9). If continuing the pregnancy is chosen, further discussions with your OB care provider and other specialists regarding the care of your baby before and after birth are important. Conversations will focus on the type of care and interventions you want to pursue. This can range from purely comfort care to partial or full **intensive intervention**. It is not uncommon for you to meet with a multidisciplinary team consisting of your obstetrician, MFM, genetic counselor or medical geneticist, neonatologist, and hopefully a perinatal palliative care specialist. A pediatric cardiologist and/or heart surgeon are helpful when a heart defect is present in the baby.

> "Decisions become acts of profound love,
> each choice a testament to the hope and heartache
> held within a parent's embrace."

Deciding on a path of pure comfort care or intensive interventions are informed by the goals that a family establishes with their care providers. We have learned from both parents and research that recognizing the goals of care for the baby before and after birth is very important and provides a road map throughout the prenatal and postnatal periods.

The common decision points include:

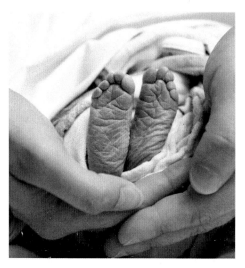

+ Fetal monitoring during labor. This would be performed to evaluate if the baby is tolerating labor.

+ Cesarean birth if the baby is in distress before or during labor or has other reasons for the procedure. These discussions can occur with your pregnancy care provider during pregnancy and prior to labor.

+ **Resuscitation** after birth in the delivery room. A newborn specialist or palliative care specialist/team are helpful in this discussion.

+ Medical and surgical interventions after birth. A family may choose full or some interventions or take a "wait and see" approach; there is much variability in how families proceed in choices surrounding care.

+ Compassionate comfort care. Support for this decision is given by a pediatric palliative care doctor, nurse, or team. Pediatric palliative care teams are increasingly available in fetal centers, children's hospitals, and neonatal intensive care units throughout the U.S. and Canada.

Families tell us that it is helpful to have discussions about these choices prior to birth. Final definite decisions do not need to be made in the first meeting and ongoing discussions are helpful.

Decisions regarding medical and surgical interventions after birth:
Recent research shows that medical and/or surgical interventions increase the chance that an infant with trisomy 18 (Edwards syndrome) will survive past the first year of life and into childhood. Interventions include:

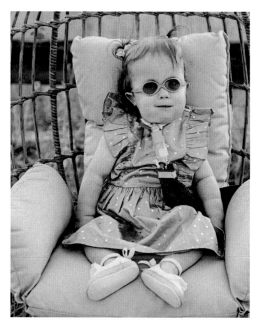

+ Oxygen adminstration

+ Respiratory technologies, such as CPAP and a ventilator to support breathing when needed

+ Feeding support such as through nasogastric(NG) tubes or gastrostomy tubes (G-tube)

+ surgeries, including cardiac surgeries to correct heart defects, tracheostomy to support breathing, or other surgeries to address concerns such as spina bifida and esophageal atresia.

Ongoing Support
Parents caring for a medically complex child tell us that there are stresses and challenges. We know that the risk for postpartum depression increases. Mental health resources are available for postpartum depression, anxiety, and depression. If needed, parents are encouraged to ask their providers for resources and services. Parents can also consider online services if that meets their needs.

PART 7: PREPARING YOUR BIRTH PLAN

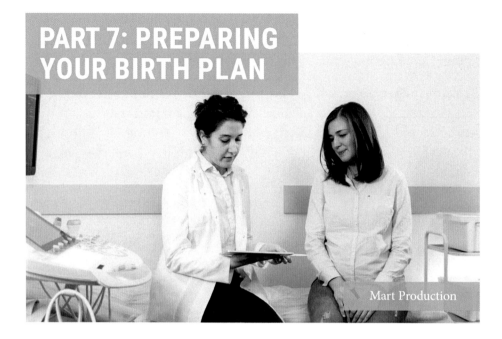

Mart Production

Having information about your baby's medical concerns and talking with your medical team can help you create a birth plan. A birth plan serves as a guide for how you envision your delivery, allowing you to consider your options and open communication with your birth team as you set care goals. While having a plan is important, it's also good to remember that sometimes babies, especially those with trisomy, have their own plans, and things may unfold differently!

"Hearing our Lukey cry when he came out of the womb brought us so much emotion: joy, relief, love, excitement."

Some of the following considerations may be limited by your pregnancy's specific health concerns and the hospital where you will be delivering. A birth plan lays out various choices at each decision landmark.

BIRTH PLAN

Parents names:

_____

Your baby's name:

_____

Name of your OB/GYN(s) and phone number(s):

_____
_____
_____
_____

Name of your baby's doctor(s) and phone number(s):

_____
_____
_____
_____

Name of important support person(s) and number(s) (friends, family, clergy, etc):

_____
_____
_____
_____

LABOR AND DELIVERY WISHES

Choose as many as you wish:
- ◯ Vaginal birth
- ◯ Cesarean birth
- ◯ Fetal heart monitoring during labor
- ◯ Who should cut umbilical cord
- ◯ Preferences for if baby is stillborn

Labor Comfort

- ○ I would like to be able to move around as I wish during labor
- ○ I would like to be able to drink fluids during labor
- ○ An intravenous (IV) line for fluids and medications
- ○ A heparin or saline lock (this device provides access to a vein but is not hooked up to a fluid bag)
- ○ A birthing ball
- ○ A birthing stool
- ○ A birthing chair
- ○ A squat bar
- ○ A warm shower or bath during delivery
- ○ Music (what type: _____)
- ○ A quiet labor room
- ○ I don't have any preferences

I would like the following people with me during labor (check hospital or birth center policy on the number of people who can be in the room):

_____

_____

It's OK [ ] It's not OK [ ] for people in training (such as medical students or residents) to be present during labor and delivery

I would like to try the following options if they are available (choose as many as you wish):

Anesthesia Options (choose one):

- ○ I do not want anesthesia offered to me during labor unless I specifically request it
- ○ I would like anesthesia. Please discuss the options with me
- ○ I do not know whether I want anesthesia. Please discuss the options with me
- ○ I prefer to avoid an episiotomy unless it is necessary

Delivery
I would like the following people with me during delivery
(check hospital or birth center policy):

_____

_____

_____

_____

For a vaginal birth

○ To use a mirror to see the baby's birth

○ For my labor partner to help support me during the pushing stage

○ For the room to be as quiet as possible

○ For one of my support people to cut the umbilical cord

○ For the lights to be dimmed

○ To be able to have one of my support people take a video or pictures of the birth

(Note: Some hospitals have policies that prohibit videotaping or taking pictures. Also, if it is allowed, the photographer needs to be positioned in a way that does not interfere with medical care)

○ For my baby to be put directly onto my chest immediately after delivery, if possible and safe to do so (please discuss any exceptions you have based on your baby's medical needs)

○ To attempt breastfeeding my baby as soon as possible after birth

○ Other: _____

For a cesarean birth

○ I would like the following person to be present with me:

_____

○ I would like one of my support people to hold the baby after delivery if I am not able to

○ I would like one of my support people to go with my baby to the nursery

○ I would like my baby to go to NICU if indicated

○ Other: _____

Medical Care

- ◯ If baby appears to be in distress, I desire a cesarean section if otherwise indicated
- ◯ We desire to have NICU in attendance for the birth
- ◯ If baby needs respiratory help we desire:
- ◯ All interventions indicated to include: oxygen supplementation, pressure support, and/or intubation if indicated
    - ◯ Only oxygen and pressure support
    - ◯ Only oxygen support
    - ◯ No intervention
- ◯ If baby is in severe distress and would otherwise need CPR, we request:
    - ◯ All interventions to include: chest compressions, IV insertion, necessary medications and fluids
    - ◯ Medications only
    - ◯ No interventions
- ◯ We desire our baby to be admitted to the NICU if otherwise required
- ◯ We desire measures such as OG, NG tubes as indicated for feeding
- ◯ We desire comfort care only
- ◯ No NICU admission. Let us have a quiet, separate room
- ◯ No invasive feeding measures such as orogastric tube, nasogastric tube, or G-tube for feeding
- ◯ We choose to be consulted and involved in all end-of-life care decisions and to ensure that our baby receives care that is consistent with comfort, dignity, and our values
- ◯ Wishes for delaying routine procedures or providing them while baby is in parent's or support person's arms

Medical Care Continued

- ○ We desire confirmation testing for Edwards syndrome
- ○ We desire all indicated consults while in the NICU
- ○ Other: _____

Feeding the Baby

Keep in mind that the baby's ability to breathe and swallow may be compromised and may require necessary interventions to support breathing and feeding.

I would like to (check as many as you wish):

- ○ Breastfeed attempts
- ○ Bottle-feed attempts
- ○ Tube feeding
- ○ A pacifier
- ○ Sugar water
- ○ Breastmilk
- ○ Formula
- ○ IV nutrition (TPN)

POST BIRTHING PLAN

We understand that our baby's condition may be life-limiting, and we are committed to ensuring that our baby receives the best possible care while maintaining comfort and quality of life.

- ◯ Would you like to go home at discharge
- ◯ Code status at discharge
- ◯ Name of support team (home health, hospice, etc) that will be assisting at home
- ◯ Anticipated needs at home
- ◯ Plan if emergency care needs arise at home
- ◯ Other: _____

Plans if baby dies before discharge
- ◯ Plans to ensure baby is comfortable during the dying process
- ◯ We desire to keep baby in room with family
- ◯ We desire for organ/tissue donation if eligible
- ◯ We desire for further testing after death
- ◯ Funeral home information
- ◯ Wishes for your child's funeral and burial arrangements
- ◯ Special wishes about transportation of baby's body
- ◯ Discuss the possibility of organ donation
- ◯ Other: _____

MEMORY MAKING

Wishes for memory-making and support
- ◯ Do you wish to have any siblings or family members involved and if so, when_____

- ○ Do you wish to have a photographer (not all hospitals have a photographer on staff)
- ○ Keepsakes: footprints, handprints, heartbeat recording, hand molds, foot molds, locks of hair, crib card, ID bands, blankets, clothing, etc
- ○ Wishes for baby and special outfits
- ○ Spiritual rituals and/or wishes to be followed during delivery and after-birth care
- ○ Other: _____

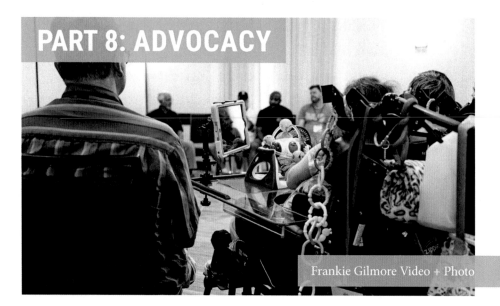

PART 8: ADVOCACY

Frankie Gilmore Video + Photo

Communicating about what you believe your baby needs can sometimes feel difficult, especially with all the information coming your way and the many decisions that need to be made. It's natural to feel overwhelmed. Medical advocacy means working with healthcare providers to gather the information you need to make the best decisions for your child's care. However, it's equally important to remember to advocate for your own emotional and mental health. Seeking support, including counseling, can be an essential part of coping with the challenges of caring for a child with complex needs. There are simple, helpful steps you can take to become a strong advocate for yourself, your family, and your baby.

+ Be aware: Learn about trisomy 18 and other conditions your child has. (see Resources, Care book, and trisomy.org)

+ Learn needs: Ask questions to learn about the specific needs your child may have and explore the available care options for each of those needs. Take time to familiarize yourself with these options and consider what may be the best fit for both your family and your child (and remember, it's okay to adjust your decisions as needed). Example: Will your baby require breathing support? Will surgery be necessary, and if so, what type(s)? Will feeding assistance be needed? Inquire about any educational classes or resources that can help you become comfortable with any equipment you may need for caring for your child at home.

- Get support: online support groups (SOFT Facebook groups) and meet in person with local trisomy families by connecting with SOFT online.

- Be assertive: This doesn't mean being aggressive, but it does mean expressing what you feel your child needs, listening to feedback, and having an open conversation with care providers. Everyone does want what is best for your child, but there may be a difference of opinion on what "best" looks like.

- Be self confident: You know your child better than anyone. You know your family better than providers. You are the best resource!

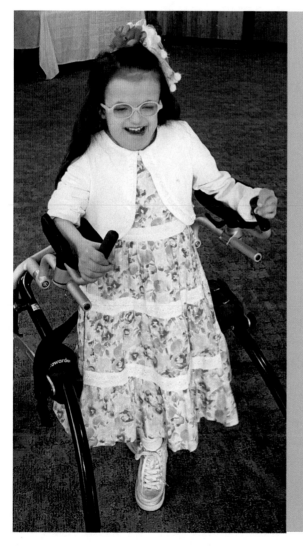

Remember your Patient Rights:
— For your needs to be met with dignity, respect, courtesy, and in a responsive and timely manner
— To receive information from your physician and have the opportunity to discuss risks and benefits of having or not having the treatment, alternative treatments, and costs
— For your physician to provide guidance about what they consider the ideal

course of action based on objective professional judgment
— To ask questions about your health, recommended treatments and to have those questions answered
— To make decisions about your care and your child's care and to have those decisions respected by the care team

— To have physicians and other staff respect your privacy and confidentiality
— To obtain copies of your medical records
— To obtain a second opinion

"Holding her for the first time. Due to her myelomeningocele surgery, we wouldn't hold her until she was healed. After 3 weeks I finally got to hold her and it is a memory I'll never forget!"

PART 9: OTHER CHOICES

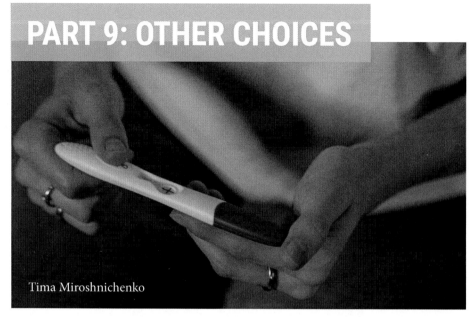

Tima Miroshnichenko

Some parents feel overwhelmed and frightened and don't know if they can do this. Every parent is different. This Part will discuss other available options.

"In the tender space between anticipation and sorrow, parents facing the birth of a trisomy baby find themselves at a crossroads where every potential path is paved with profound love, deep reflection, and the quiet strength of cherishing each moment given"

Pregnancy Termination/Abortion

After receiving a prenatal diagnosis and learning about trisomy 18, some parents will choose to terminate the pregnancy. An obstetric provider, medical geneticist, or genetic counselor can provide safe options for termination in your area or surrounding region. Abortion care has changed rapidly in the U.S. since 2022, so it is crucial that you understand the current laws in your state. This may mean traveling to a different state for the termination. At this time, restriction is based largely on gestational age/presence of a heart beat.

As a general rule, termination is typically safer the earlier it can be performed. Most commonly, pregnancies with a baby with a chromosome condition are not diagnosed and confirmed until late first trimester or in the second trimester, which may limit a family's options regarding termination in their state.

There are two basic modes of termination: medical and surgical. Medical termination involves the administration of particular medicines that cause an abortion; it is done in the first trimester usually by 10 weeks and can often be performed as an outpatient. Surgical termination, particularly in the second trimester, is performed by a procedure called dilation and evacuation (D&E) and is done as an in-patient.

The issue of mental health and pregnancy termination is complex and research can be conflicting. As with any person receiving unexpected news, it is important to consider utilizing mental health resources for help both during and after the process. Because pregnancy termination can be associated with depression and other reactions, some women will appreciate referral to supportive resources.

Adoption
It is possible for birth parents to choose to place their child for adoption. There are families that seek out adopting children with trisomy 18 (Edwards syndrome).

> "We chose to adopt a child with Edwards syndrome because he has so much love to share and is a huge blessing to our lives."

The first step when making the decision to place a child for adoption is to talk with a social worker and an adoption agency. The second step is to choose the adoptive family. You will need to share as much medical information as you have about the child to ensure that the adopting family is prepared for all that the child will need. You also need to decide the amount of involvement you want with the family for the remainder of your pregnancy and also with the family after the child is born.

RESOURCES

www.trisomy.org

Care Book
https://trisomy.org/resources/parenting-a-child
/care-book-trisomy-18-trisomy-13/#/

MEDICAL REFERENCES

PART 1 & 2

- Screening for fetal chromosomal abnormalities. ACOG Practice Bulletin No. 226. American College of Obstetricians and Gynecologists. Obstet Gynecol 2020;136:e48–69.

- Indications for outpatient antenatal fetal surveillance. ACOG Committee Opinion No. 828. American College of Obstetricians and Gynecologists. Obstet Gynecol 2021;137:e177–97.

- Antepartum fetal surveillance. ACOG Practice Bulletin No. 229. American College of Obstetricians and Gynecologists. Obstet Gynecol 2021;137:e116–27.

- Second-trimester abortion. Practice Bulletin No. 135. American College of Obstetricians and Gynecologists. Obstet Gynecol 2013;121:1394–1406.

PART 3

- Carey JC. Perspectives on the care and management of infants with trisomy 18 and trisomy 13: striving for balance. Curr Opin Pediatr 2012, 24: 672-678.

- Cortezzo DE, Tolusso LK, Swarr DT. Perinatal Outcomes of Fetuses and Infants diagnosed with trisomy 13 or 18. J of Pediatr, 2022, 247:116-123.e5. doi: 10.1016/j.jpeds.2022.04.010

- Genetics Home Reference https://medlineplus.gov/genetics/condition/trisomy-18/Genet

- Haug S, Goldstein M, Cummins D, Fayard E, Merritt TA. Using patient centered care after a prenatal diagnosis of trisomy 18 or trisomy 13: a review. JAMAPediatrics 2017, 171:382-387.

MEDICAL REFERENCES

PART 3 CONTINUED

- Lorenz JM and Hardart GE. Evolving medical and surgical management of infants with trisomy 18. Curr Opin Pediatr 2014, 26:169-176.

- Weaver MS, Anderson V, Beck J, Delaney JW, Ellis C, Fletcher S, et al. Interdisciplinary care of children with trisomy 13 and 18. American Journal of Medical Genetics Part A 2021, 185A:966-977.

PART 7

- https://www.ama-assn.org/delivering-care/ethics/patient-rights#:~:text=To%20courtesy%2C%20respect%2C%20 dignity%2C,and%20costs%20of%20forgoing%20treatment.

- https://www.childrenscolorado.org/conditions-and-advice/ parenting/parenting-articles/advocating-for-your-child/

- https://adc.bmj.com/content/101/7/596

- https://blog.cincinnatichildrens.org/rare-and-complex-conditions/ advocating-for-your-child-some-practical-suggestions/

MEDICAL REFERENCES

PART 8

⊕ Reardon DC. The abortion and mental health controversy: A comprehensive literature review of common ground agreements, disagreements, actionable recommendations, and research opportunities. SAGE Open Med. 2018 Oct 29;6:2050312118807624. doi: 10.1177/2050312118807624. PMID: 30397472; PMCID: PMC6207970.

GLOSSARY

AMNIOCENTESIS — a prenatal diagnostic technique where a needle is placed into the uterus and a small amount of amniotic fluid is withdrawn usually for performing testing

BIRTH DEFECTS — congenital abnormalities of the structure of organs or body parts

CHORIONIC VILLUS SAMPLING (CVS) — a prenatal diagnostic technique where a small amount of placental tissue (chorionic villus) is taken for performing testing

CHROMOSOME — threadlike structures seen only by microscope in the nucleus of cells and carrying the genes

ECHOCARDIOGRAM — an ultrasound study of the heart, if prenatal a fetal echocardiogram

EDWARDS SYNDROME — the pattern of physical findings and differences originally described by Dr John Edwards in 1960 and caused by trisomy 18

FETAL CENTER — multidisciplinary teams recently established in the U.S and Canada to help manage complex pregnancies especially those with fetuses with birth defects

FETUS — developing baby in the womb before birth

GENE — the fundamental unit of heredity and made up of specific DNA

INTENSIVE INTERVENTION — Medical treatment that is meant to prolong life, including ventilators and surgeries

MOSAICISM — 2 or more genetically different cell lines in a person

NONINVASIVE PRENATAL SCREENING (NIPS) — maternal blood sample obtained at 10-11 weeks gestation to study cell- free DNA derived from the fetus

POSITIVE PREDICTIVE VALUE (PPV) — the chance that a positive result of a screening test will predict a condition, for example, trisomy 18

RESUSCITATION — process or act of reviving or correcting difficulties in an acutely ill person

STILLBIRTH — a fetus (baby in the womb) of greater than 20 weeks of pregnancy who dies in the womb prior to birth

SYNDROME — a recognizable pattern of multiple birth defects

TRANSLOCATION — an exchange of chromosomal material between 2 chromosomes

TRISOMY — an extra copy of a chromosome

TRISOMY 18 — 3 copies of the # 18 chromosome and the cause of Edwards syndrome

ULTRASOUND — a procedure using sound waves to look at tissues and organs; also called a sonogram

TRISOMY 18
New and Expectant Parent Resource Guide

Prepared By Support Organization for Trisomy 18, 13, and Related Disorders (SOFT)

SOFT CONTRIBUTERS:
John C. Carey MD, MPH
Kelly Hernandez M.Ed, M.Sp
Kris Holladay
Terre Krotzer
Jennifer L. H. Sogge MD
Terra L. Spiehs-Garst RN, MSN, CLC
Barb VanHerreweghe
Jacqueline Vidosh MD

Special thanks to Nick Holladay,
SOFT Director of Technology

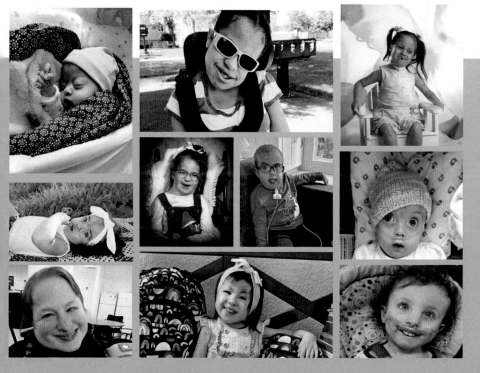

Made in United States
Orlando, FL
17 December 2024

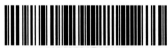

56069528R00027